A guide for
The Nurse Entrepreneur

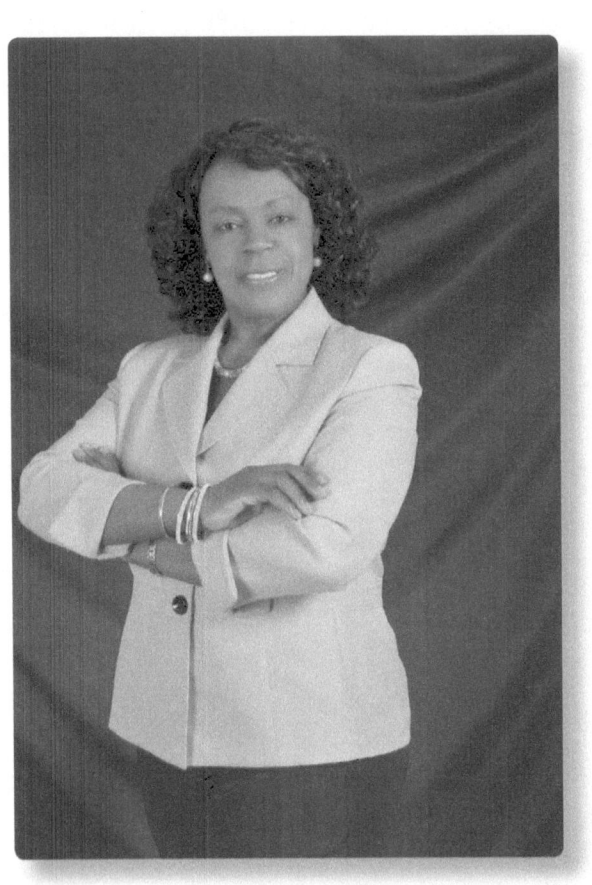

A guide for
The Nurse Entrepreneur

Make a Difference

EMPOWER – ENGAGE – INSPIRE

Eva M. Francis RN,MSN,CCRN

To order additional copies of this book, contact:
Xlibris
1-888-795-4274
www.Xlibris.com
Orders@Xlibris.com
615563

Liability Notice

A guide to Nurse Entrepreneur is for informational purposes only. The ideas, suggestions, general principles, and conclusions presented here reflect the views of the author, and your implementation of the information provided can be used and be adapted to fit your own particular situation or circumstance.

The author/publisher has made every effort to ensure the accuracy of the information herein. However, the information contained in this guide is provided without warranty, either expressed or implied. Your use of any information contained in this property can be made available on EvaMfrancis.com and used at your own risk.

Table of Contents

Acknowledgment

This is my second print book, and I would like to dedicate it to my extraordinary parents, who I consider my super heroes. Mr. Vincent Francis (he is ninety-two years young at the time of writing this book), and the late Mrs. Eunice Francis, who both believed that I could be all that I was designed to be, even when others questioned my life's goals. These two individuals have been my rock over the years not only with their children, but also with all other children in and for that I am forever grateful for their love, their patience and their kindness. I also want to thank them for their unwavering dedication, and support over the years with not only me, but also all other children in our small community of MT Pleasant, St Catherine, Jamaica West Indies

I dedicate this book with deep admiration and praise to them. It is so fitting when others in the community chose to label them matriarch and patriarch of the great community. You both did your best with all your children and could not have done it any better. Your excellence as parents will continue to shine and radiate in my life. I love and appreciate you both for all the lives that you have touched and all the impact that you have made in the lives that you have come in contact with. I will confidently say that you are the best. Thank you from the bottom of my heart and I am forever grateful.

Introduction

The purpose of this book is to allow nurses as well as other healthcare professionals to understand as well as learn of many of the alternatives that are available to them, so that they can recondition their thinking, as they grow in their nursing career regardless of the path or the journey that they choose.

I also want to give health-care professionals particular nurses a glimpse of other areas that they can embrace as they seek ways to make a greater impact through entrepreneurship.

Chapter 1

The Healthcare Landscape

He who has health has hope and He who has hope has
everything- Anonymous-

Continuing Healthcare Industry Changes:
Impact on Nursing Profession

The healthcare system is adapting to the ever-changing needs and demands of healthcare users. Over the last decades, there has been significant changes in how healthcare is delivered particularly a shift to a more preventive approach. There have been transitions for those in the nursing profession that have promised to change the practice of nurses, expand upon current nursing roles, make room for new nursing roles, and provide several opportunities for nurses to participate in molding the future delivery system of health care. The health-care industry is facing unprecedented challenges, and nurses as well as other healthcare professionals must brace themselves to play a major role in meeting them.

Since the Affordable Care Act (ACA) was passed in 2010, care delivery and financing systems have been undergoing major changes that are continuing to accelerate and evolve. Due to the ACA, millions more Americans have, and will continue to gain access to healthcare as well as having and owning health insurance. Therefore, this will require a sizable workforce to meet the increased demand for care. This increased demand for care is causing the health-care workforce to be faced with the burden of stress and instability because a major redesign of health-care providers will be needed to accommodate the care needed for millions more of Americans.

One goal that stems from the ACA is for enhanced coverage for preventative care services to help shift the current focus of the delivery system. The current focus is on acute care; however, this needs to be shifted to having a greater emphasis on prevention and treatment of chronic conditions using health-care teams along with information technology.

With the continuing advancements of technology and the aging human population, the challenges nurses face remains daunting and are not getting much easier. The health conditions that individuals are diagnosed with are becoming more chronic, requiring longer duration of treatment, as well as any necessary adjustments in treatment based on the unfamiliar route that many conditions decide to take. We frequently hear about new strains of illnesses surfacing or diseases becoming resistant to current treatments. This requires the nursing profession to break out of it's comfort zone and embrace new ways to provide treatment and care. Some nurses may opt to continue and advance their education so that they may increase their level of practice for certain situations.

Another impact that the ever-changing health-care industry may have on the nursing profession is causing shortages of medical professionals, an issue that is especially predominant in rural areas. Along with an aging population, we also have an aging workforce that is going to cause hundreds of thousands, or even millions, of job openings for nurses and physicians within the next decade. In conjunction with the numerous new additions to the medical profession, there will be new attitudes toward professional roles and responsibilities that differ from those of the prior generation that held these positions. There will most likely not be enough licensed nursing professionals in the United States to take care of the number of Americans that will be using the expected new health-care system based on current trends. This is scary to think about because if there are not enough professionals to handle the aging population and their chronic conditions, it may result in increased morbidity and mortality, especially for rural Americans. With a health-care-professional shortage and possible increases in mortality, this would defeat the goal of prevention to increase the lifespan and quality of life. How do we combat such shortage? Organizations in the US will opt to the international healthcare market.

More and more, patients are entering the health-care setting just because they are now insured via the Affordable Care Act. This results in a heavier workload for the professionals taking care of them, followed by more stress, more paperwork, longer hours, more errors, and fatigue. Ultimately, this can lead to fatigue, becoming burned out or second-guessing their career decision. I suppose the optimistic person would view this as there being only one way to go from the current health-care-industry situation, and that is up! However, to push past the long hours, heavy workloads, prolonged dissatisfaction, and increased stress, one must be stretched to their limits and be 100 percent passionate about their career. It always seems that if you stick with something long enough, the positive aura of it seems to shine through sooner or later.

In this day and age, year after year and with advancement after advancement, we all need to do our best to accept the changes in the health-care industry and hope that the kinks work themselves out. The majority of the changes can be beneficial if carried out correctly, especially in medicine. Embrace the changes as best as you possibly can because it could mean a cure for your disease or adding a few more years to your life to spend with those you love.

After the passing of the ACA in 2010, care delivery and financing systems have been undergoing major changes that are continuing to accelerate. Due to the ACA, millions more Americans have gained, and are going to continue to gain, health insurance; therefore, this will require a sizable workforce to meet the increased demand for care. This increased demand for care is causing the health-care workforce to be faced with the burden of stress and instability because a major redesign of health-care providers is needed to accommodate the care needed for millions more of Americans. One goal that stems from the ACA is for enhanced coverage for preventative care services to help shift the current focus of the delivery system. The current focus is on acute care; however, this focus needs to be shifted to put a greater emphasis on prevention and treatment of chronic conditions using health-care teams along with information technology.

I write about health care with the same passion that I have in caring for patients and families. That is my passion, my gift, and I love it.

Recently, I read a great article from Forbes Magazine that states, "[The] Healthcare Industry must reinvent itself using Leadership from the Business World." As I read the article, I began to learn, or rather it dawned on me that as leaders, we have a great responsibility to lock ourselves into whatever transition is taking place. That is the only way we are going to be equipped to lead the next generation in caring for patients and their families.

The health-care industry is one of the largest and fastest-growing industries in the United States, and with the increase in retiring baby boomers, health-care professionals are looking for ways that they can grow, change jobs, or seek an alternative to the traditional occupations. This applies to nurses, along with other allied health professionals such as case managers, pharmacists, etc. I thought long and hard and decided to write about this ever-changing landscape of "the great health-care industry."

I can remember so many great stories about the health-care industry and the lives that have been touched over the years. Being in this career for so long, I have seen the best of this industry and I also seen some undesirable aspects of the industry as well. One of the things I admire most about health care is the ability to make a great impact on people and add value to their lives. Not only do you touch the lives of patients every day, but you also touch the lives of their families and loved ones. The health-care system is undergoing a dramatic transformation, and there is a huge focus on the Affordable Care Act, which results in an increased number of patients seeking health care. Given this, there is a push to surviving in the new economy. With this in mind, health-care professionals cannot overlook the fact that a reinvention in career may be necessary.

I have a friend who worked as a guest relation officer in her organization for a number of years; however, as her industry experienced changes, she was laid off. After she went through the initial phases of denial, shock, and acceptance, she decided to reinvent herself and start her own customer service training company. She is now a customer service strategist in her company, and her business has grown and will soon be a multimillion-dollar corporation.

Believe it or not, there is someone out there who wants what you have, and in addition, each of us have a specific and unique gift to offer. Perhaps one of my mentors put it best, "We must start before we are ready, and build the plan while we start."

Why Healthcare Entrepreneurship

In today's health-care industry, there have been some notable changes taking place, and consequently, there have been an equal number of entrepreneurial opportunities and activities as a direct response to the changes taking place. The health-care economy is a trillion-dollar economy. Governments around the world have increased spending on health care, and individuals understand that for a government to run properly, health care is not luxury but, rather, an obligation.

According to Forbes Magazine, in 2014 alone, there has been a vast increase in the number of start-ups involved in the health-care industry, such as Omaha Health, which connects those at risk for chronic diseases like diabetes to a comprehensive lifestyle-change program that includes a personal health coach and a digital support group. Venture capitalists are spending billions of dollars in the industry, as much as $4.1 billion in Silicon Valley, according to a report on CNBC. There is a wealth of support for entrepreneurs who are developing new solutions to address some of the growing pains in health care.

Entrepreneurs involved in the health-care industry help aid the current providers of health-care services by introducing innovative technologies that in many cases make it easier to do their job. This, however, does not mean that becoming an entrepreneur in the health-care industry is easy. Entrepreneurship in any industry is not easy, as not everyone can be an entrepreneur. There are many reasons to become an entrepreneur; specifically, for the health-care sector, the benefits are the following:

Increase investment—one of the main reasons that entrepreneurs should consider health-care entrepreneurship is the amount of funds being pumped into the sector by venture capitalists. As previously stated, there has been a record increase in the amount of money start-ups are receiving for their ideas.

Opportunity—There are plenty of opportunities involved in the health-care industry; this helps explain why there is so much money being pumped into it.

Social responsibility—Some of the opportunities that are present in the health-care industry are as a result of many medical practitioners and other entrepreneurs' commitment to help build and improve their society.

Make a difference in people's lives—the most successful entrepreneurs are the ones that set out first to make a difference as opposed to make money. Health is one of the best places that entrepreneurs can do something to help effect real change in people's lives. In many cases when the primary objective for an entrepreneurial undertaking is, in fact, to effect change, money and financial freedom always follow.

In many cases in the health-care industry, doctors and health-care practitioners are the ones getting involved in entrepreneurship, though savvy entrepreneurs who are not doctors are normally able to identify the opportunities involved and take advantage of them. Health care is becoming, and will remain, a great opportunity hub for entrepreneurship. It is estimated that in 2015, more health-care start-ups will emerge, and more venture capitalists will invest money in these companies. The time for health-care entrepreneurship is now, and more smart entrepreneurs will indeed be getting involved in this industry.

Questions to Ask Yourself before or during the First Days of Your Business

Is this business a good idea?

Is this a product or service worth buying? Will this product or service change the lives of individuals? Are you going to turn a profit or be in the red? Do the math.

Do you have a "WHY?" "WHATS YOUR WHY?"

Why are you starting a business? Understand that when the challenges come knocking at your door, you must go back to the "WHY" Your why will help you through the dark times which every entrepreneur face. Your "Why" will take you through the highs and the lows, and there are lessons to be learned from both.

Do you have a business plan?

Yes, you need one. Make it clear and be as detailed as possible, but know that it may need to be changed in the future as your business adapts to the consumers.

Can you be in it for the long haul?

Businesses don't pop up overnight. Profits come even later. Have a reliable money source while your business gets going. Do you have money saved up? Can your spouse, family or loved ones support you? Don't put off looking into financing if you need it.

Does your family support you?

Think of your family as your first customers. You need to convince them that your product/service is profitable. If they're on your side, it will make all other challenges easier.

What's the company name?

Make it memorable, but make sure it's new. Use the Internet and search the names to make sure it isn't taken at state or federal level.

Have you registered the domain name, and are you online?

And no, it shouldn't be yourbusiness@yahoo.com. You need to show your customers that you are the authentic and that you've invested in this. Make a website for your business, even if you aren't fully up and running. Everything is on the Internet, and customers see it as a way to verify you.

Will you become Social?

Make a Facebook Page. Yes, Facebook, LinkedIn and Twitter. Social media is a way to reach your customers as well as spread the word of your business. Make sure you build your brand with your business name. Knowem.com is a good way to reserve your name and business cards. They aren't expensive, and they give you a credibility boost.

Have you applied for an EIN?

Getting an employer identification number (EIN) makes sure you aren't the same as your business. Plus, you'll need an EIN if you want to incorporate or have a bank account for your business. It's free.

Have you registered for a business bank account?

It's easy in the beginning to charge everything personally but difficult to untangle later. Don't create a tangle. Create a separate account, with an accounting system. Keep the books in order. Messy books are a messy business.

Have you incorporated, and is the paperwork done?

Meet with your attorney and accountant to talk about the legal issues of business. Incorporating can be a big help. Also, you may need more than one business license, depending on what your business is. Make sure you look into licenses—the SBA is helpful—and get all that you need.

Also, depending on your business, you may need customer contracts. Have your lawyer create them. You may need patents too. Those can come a little later.

Have you got the space?

Have you got a brick-and-mortar business? If so, get your space now. Are you running retail? Think about foot traffic and how accessible everything is. But if you don't have either brick-and-mortar or retail, hold off on the space. You don't need to add lease payments on top of your already-growing expenses in starting a business.

Do you have cofounders, and do they have jobs?

Who is doing what? Talk about it, agree on it, and write it down. Make sure everyone is clear in what they are doing. You need to stay united. A house divided cannot stand.

Now that the really important tasks are done, you can wait a while before you do all these. But don't put them off too long!

Do you have a good pitch?

If you have a good elevator pitch, you can attract all sorts of important people to your business: business partners, investors, employees, and most importantly, customers. You need to have a clear pitch to pull people in. As you go along, use customer feedback to make sure this pitch is always current.

Do you need help? Ask for it.

Find someone who has a successful business in the same area as yours. Ask for help. They have been through what you are experiencing. They can give you advice and help you talk through ideas.

Is your business insured?

You're likely going to need some sort of insurance, whether it be health insurance or worker's comp. Talk to your insurance agent.

Have you started hiring your staff?

If you work in a business that needs staff from day one, get started on this sooner. But otherwise, you may be able to use interns and freelancers at first. Just make sure that you have some sort of help. You can't be a one-person business. You need some kind of help. You can start out as chief salesperson, but you need a sales team that can function without you so you can focus on other aspects of the business.

Have you got everything you need?

If you're going into retail or manufacturing, you need a supply to be selling. Make sure you have a reliable supply. Confirm that all services, like phone and Internet and the like, are secured as well. If you're using computers or other devices, make sure you have an IT service to protect your data.

OTHERS QUESTIONS TO ASK YOURSELF

Are there competitors? If so, who and where are they?

Is this going to make me feel better than I feel right now?

What is the viability of my idea? Is this lucrative?

What do I have a passion for?

What is my secret "sauce" in health care?

What are my nurse and/or health-care specialties?

What are my natural talents? Maybe teaching, coaching, training, inventions, writing, etc.

This checklist is not the end-all, be-all, but it helps you get your priorities in order. Make your own checklist to make starting your own business seem less overwhelming.

Chapter 2

My Journey into Nursing

A man can succeed at almost anything for which he has unlimited enthusiasm.
—Charles Schwab

Many times I look back at my career journey and ask myself, what would I change if I had to start the journey all over again? It is hard to decide what to change. I am grateful that I worked many of my nursing years in places where nursing is considered a desirable profession. Early in my nursing career, I made a decision that I had no choice but to love it. My parents had ten children, and it is typical for a traditional Jamaican family to decide a career track for you. As a little girl growing up, I was called nurse by the community members so very early in life, I knew that I was going to be a nurse. I started my nursing career in 1978.

Thirty years ago, I graduated from the School of Nursing at the University of the West Indies, Kingston, Jamaica, and what a journey it has been. I had the opportunity to work at so many different places: hospitals, community centers, academic medical centers, community-based organizations, prisons, rural villages, urban slums, and from the bedside to the boardroom. I must say that my experience has been more than wonderful.

The gift and calling of the nursing profession have fueled me to walk my path. This is a journey that, I must say, I have enjoyed to the very maximum. However, I cannot deny that I have met many roadblocks along the way. Many tears were shed, and there were many moments of joy and appreciation. My journey has allowed me to meet, talk with, care for, laugh with, and be present with different people over the years, and this has been one of the most rewarding parts of my life. You tend to grow when you are not restricted to your comfort zone; often, it is in those uncomfortable or difficult spaces that we truly see ourselves. This is the life and people that sometimes exist in the shadows. It is easy to ignore the shadows, easy to not see the disparities, inequities, and the overt world of the "haves" and the "have-nots", anywhere around the globe. It can be ugly; it can be hard to not be in the majority, to be the one that is different. Some of you know these challenges all too well.

Chapter 3

Passion for Patient Care

If you can't figure out your purpose, figure out your passion. For your passion will lead you right into your purpose – Bishop T D Jakes -

As I excelled in the career of nursing, I realized that I have a deep passion to care, and I lived the mission of providing the best possible care for patients. My belief is that patients and families must be empowered to provide for own their health, and at the same time, they deserve the right to receive the best possible care. It is always my philosophy that we should bring out the best of us as nurses.

I have seen great nurses, and I have seen some who are burned out still forcing themselves to stay in their current position. I believe, if you reach the stage where you no longer are able to provide the best care for a patient, then it is time to reconsider or reinvent yourself.

When I made the decision to reinvent myself and embark on the transition from the hospital walls to launching my own business, I was not burned out, stressed, or bitter. I just felt it was time for me to pursue my passion and my calling while I still unleashed my nursing and health-care brilliance to touch lives indirectly. I wanted to make my own schedule and be more creative and expressive with my talents while sharing my talents and experiences in a big way. I wanted to have more time for myself, family, and church and take more vacations without having to worry about going back to work tired after a vacation. I also wanted to wake up without an alarm clock and not work all hours of the day (or night). Of course, I also wanted more money, but this was not, should not, be the main reason.

This is the best decision that I have made for myself thus far. Now I am so happy. I am at peace spiritually, financially, mentally, physically, and emotionally.

Chapter 4

Reinvention Strategies

Our job as nurses is to cushion the sorrow, and celebrate the joy, every day while we are just doing our jobs.
—Christine Bell

Reinvention

Are you ready to reinvent your calling and career?

Are you ready to elevate yourself and increase your level of living?

Are you ready to touch lives in a bigger way?

Are you ready to make a bigger impact in the world?

Are you ready for financial freedom?

Are you ready to unleash your God-given brilliance?

Are you finally ready to launch your business?

Let us talk about reinvention: As time goes by in life, we all need to step back and reinvent ourselves in one area of our lives or another. Reinvention does not necessarily mean to "make a change in behavior." It means a little more than that.

When we speak of reinvention, it is not like you are just "polishing up yourself" or improving yourself or simply making things a bit better. I'm talking about the reset button (life's button, by taking things to another level). Reinvention is a change in what you believe and how you do your job. If you are up for the challenge, then you can start now. You can do this. How? Do the work that matters.

Synonyms to the word reinvention, according to the thesaurus, are the following:

Revamp

Renew

Remake

Refresh

Revive

Restore

Resuscitate

Reproduce

These words are available to anyone; they are available to you if you want them. No matter what is going on in the economy, we can use it as an opportunity to make a difference, spread our ideas, and make an impact. Many of us who are fortunate to be in the HealthCare industry and are health-care profession have more leverage, more chances, and more power to change the world now than any other time in history.

How Do You Know When It Is Time to Reinvent?

You know it is time to reinvent yourself when you . . .

No longer enjoy your job,

Do not feel like going to work,

Are taking more sick days than you are actually sick,

Are constantly late for work,

Do not care about the patients and their families,

Know patients and their families are no longer top priority,

Begin saying things like "I am just here to take care of my patients,"

Feel overly stressed and/or burned out,

Start to make mistakes, medication errors, and complain about government mandates,

Are already in a leadership role,

No longer part of the solution for the company,

No longer provide top quality care and compassion.

If you fit in any of the above-referenced categories, then it is probably time for you to reset your career button and reinvent yourself.

My definition of reinvention is to "recreate, start fresh, renew, regenerate, and revitalize yourself!" All of which I had to do when I decided to leave the hospital as a nurse and go back as a business owner in the health-care field.

So What Alternatives Are There? Nurse Entrepreneurship

Nursing entrepreneurship provides nurses with self-employment opportunities, which allow them to pursue their personal vision and passion to improve health outcomes using innovative approaches. Similar to other entrepreneurs, a nurse entrepreneur is considered to be a "proprietor of a business that offers nursing services of a direct care, educational, research, administrative, or consultative nature." There are many opportunities and business ideas out there for nurses and other health-care professionals.

Nurses comprise a large proportion of the health-care workforce and are considered to be the frontline staff across the health continuum in most health services and countries. In spite of the immense and significant role that nurses play in the health-care system, they are seldom considered equal partners in multidisciplinary health-care teams. As a result, the unique skills held by generalist and specialist nurses are often underutilized and even, at times, undervalued across the health continuum.

Many nurses want to do their best, but because of various reasons in the health-care system, nurses at times are stuck in a rut that they cannot seem to get out of. It is paramount that they get out and continue to give care and enjoy success.

The Reinvention Process

Reinvention does not necessarily mean that you must walk away from the bedside. Sometimes you may need to change your location, your specialty, and/or your health-care provider. You need to get more education to advance yourself.

While the reinvention process is different for everyone, I am going to be focusing on the entrepreneurial alternatives and business ideas for health-care workers specifically.

The main thing is, whenever you get an idea, write it down. Write everything down. It is a known as a "brain dump" and will become very useful in later steps. When it comes to owning your business, you must be specific. I cannot overemphasize the importance of clarity.

When you decide to be a business owner, you must be clear on exactly why you want to be. If your reason is driven by money, then I highly suggest that you reconsider. The reason has to be more solid and concrete, such as spending more time with your family.

Continuing Education

Recently, someone asked me about continuing education, "Is it a viable business? And why nurses would pay for continuing education when so much was being offered for free?"

These are great questions. Too often I hear of nurses who have started an entrepreneur business without first determining if there is an eager, excited market ready to buy what they have to offer. One way to determine if there is a market for your services is to look around and see if anyone else is offering the same or similar product or service.

In the area of nursing continuing education, there are companies offering nursing continuing education training. It may or may not be a lucrative idea. You will need to determine what makes your company unique and how you will compete.

What Would Make You Special?

The next question to answer would be "Why do nurses buy continuing education?" Some employers may pay for continuing education to help the nurses stay current with their education or as a retention benefit.

Some nurses may not have continuing education covered by their employers, but they still need it for their licensure, so they purchase it themselves. While there are many continuing education units that are offered for free, nurses may still decide to purchase continuing education from a company. Reasons for purchasing continuing education vary from nurse to nurse. Some nurses have no choice but to pay because their company may not be approved by a particular state for licensure requirements or for a specific certifying body. There are also nurses who prefer that the education they receive is evidence-based, and they may want to pay to get access to that type of training.

One of the best ways to determine why nurses pay for continuing education is to find some nurses who have been paying and ask them why they choose to pay for this education.

The above are just a few examples, but there are so many more ideas out there.

What to Know Before You Start

After you establish the why you want to start your own business, you must research your business idea for viability. The Nurse Entrepreneur

Network website is a great resource to start your research on verifying the viability of your nurse entrepreneur product or service: http://www.nurse-entrepreneur-network.com/.

Next, figure out who or what your target market is. Identify the types of people you wish to have as your customers. List as many characteristics as you can about these people, such as age, gender, occupation, income level, interests, education, lifestyle, and anything else you can think of that is specific to your ideal customer. Who is your ideal target, and can they afford to pay for your services?

Confirm if there are enough potential customers in your ideal client group to support your business. Be sure you know where your potential clients might gather. If you cannot find where they gather, you will not be able to sell effectively enough to sustain your business.

If you are a speaker or a coach, you need to have your topics outlined. You need to know the material and how to present it.

You need to figure out how to connect with your target market. You need to build your network and socialize with your target audience.

The Three Most Important Components for Nurse Entrepreneurs to Get Noticed on the Internet

To get noticed as a nurse entrepreneur, there are a couple of critical things you can do. You want to establish yourself as a nurse entrepreneur expert and be able to be found. The three most important components for doing this are thus:

Create a website—as a nurse entrepreneur, you need to be able to be found. Having a website is an important part of making it easy for clients to find you as well as your products and services. You must have contact information on your site, including your name, business name, business address, telephone number, and e-mail address. Make it easy for your potential customers to find and contact you.

Start and contribute to a blog and/or group—by creating a blog or group, you have a place where you can regularly post quality information. I have a blog, a Facebook business page, and a LinkedIn group. In this instance, more is better. You have more places to post information that may be accessed by different types of people, and you can have more external links going to your website, which helps your page ranking in Google and other search engines. The content you post should be valuable content that will be perceived as helpful by your target audience. This helps you become recognized as a nurse entrepreneur expert. Posting content is one of the best ways for your target audience to get to "know, like, and trust" you. Your target audience is not likely to buy from you until they feel that they know, like, and trust you. Make it easy for them to feel comfortable with you by giving a lot of useful and actionable information.

Participate in social media sites—read and post in sites like Facebook, LinkedIn, and Twitter. Joining sites where your target audience can be reached is a great way to get your name out there. After joining, you can respond to questions and post information that will be helpful for your target market. These sites are also an excellent place to discover the challenges of your target audience. You can learn what you should be creating by reading about the questions your target market is asking, writing about, and commenting on. Mind these sites for topics for your next postings.

Build on these components to establish yourself as a nurse entrepreneur expert. They will go a long way in helping you get noticed among all the traffic on the Internet.

Keys to Success When You Get Started

Be consistent with everything. Whether it is advertising, blogging, fliers, all promotional material should be consistent. Build your brand awareness. Keep your images, colors, and so on consistent.

Throughout your business venture, always remember why you are doing this in the first place. Is it because you want to help people? Are you making a difference in other people's lives? Is it your passion?

The message that I want to leave with you is this:

Reinvent your calling and your career in nursing and health care. The world is waiting to see what you can bring to the table. Live, dream, and teach to a higher purpose. Care with integrity, give with intensity, and have compassion and sensitivity. Lead your team with vision, passion, and purpose. Your destiny is waiting to manifest, so provide clarity to your destiny and purpose to your mission.

I have a little story to share about a fellow nurse I knew. For the purpose of this writing, I will call her Nurse J. She became a nurse sixteen years ago while she was raising a family. She considers herself a front line RN because she spent most of her clinical years working in an emergency department. She worked very hard and enjoyed her work immensely. She enjoyed taking care of patients, and she even felt like nursing was her gift as well as her calling. Each and every day, she felt validated that nursing was her passion and she was indeed making a huge difference in the lives of others. However, as time came to pass, according to her, working for the same company was no longer an enjoyment because she was "carved to fit." My advice to Nurse J and to those of you who are reading this book is to reevaluate your life and be truthful to yourself. Only you have the power to make yourself happy. The very virtue of the word nurse is to care for others; do not forsake that caregiving can manifest itself in different forms. Being a nurse on a reinvented platform can be the key to your success and the catalyst to performing your call to duty on an entirely different level.

Chapter 5

Alternatives to Bedside Nursing
/ the Idea Factory

Below are fifty different ways to manifest your call of duty to be a nurse.

Health-care organizational consultant

Health-care professional speaker

Health-care motivational speaker

Health-care holistic coach

Health and wellness coach

Health integrative coach

Legal nurse consultant

Health and fitness coach

Health-care training-center business

Hosting seminars and workshops

Nurse informatics consultant

Health-care software consultant

Nursing career, résumé writing, and nursing interview consultant

Nursing weight-loss business

Stress management coach for health-care professionals

Executive nurse leader, coach, and consultant

NCLEX training for nurses' business

CPR, AED, first aid training business

Online writing for health-care website and marketers

Adult day care center

Child day care services

Ghostwriting for medical profession

Medical inventor

Companion care business

Private duty independent business

Staffing agency business

Health-care author and writer

Health-care advocacy

Affordable Care Act and health-care reform training business

Critical care and emergency services training business

Continuing education business

Certified nursing assistant training center

Nurse informatics business and basic computer business

Home health agency business

ALF business

Nursing school business

Nursing home business

Health-care marketing business

Creating first aid kits business

Medical software programs business

Alternative health-care center (such as aromatics herbal treatment)

Doula services (assisting laboring mothers)

Natural-childbirth class

Online medical information center

Launching community health fairs

Medical braces business (assisting people with injuries)

Medical equipment and medical cushions sales

Mobile hearing testing

Vitamin sales business

Home care education for quality measures in hospitals

I.   Ensuring that you truly want to own your own business

II.   What kind of business (consider your passions, knowledge, experience, credentials, and licensures)

III. Office space or home-based business

IV.   Seeking a coach or a mentor

V.   Branding, including website and business cards

VI.   Social media

VII. Marketing

VIII. Contracts and legal implications

IX.   Prices

Nurses are unique professionals. Each of you has a lot to offer to the world, so do it with all you might. If you decide to be a health-care professional or a motivational speaker, the world is waiting to hear you. The world is waiting for what you have to offer. Live and reach for your highest purpose. Try to do something beyond what you thought you could do. Do not be afraid to step out of your comfort zone. Do not be afraid to shine and do what you do best. Lead with vision, passion, and purpose. Your potential, your true self, and your destiny are waiting to manifest. Provide clarity to your destiny and purpose to your nursing mission.

Give with intensity, care, sensitivity, and integrity. I applaud each of you for the giving of yourself daily. Whether you give care directly or indirectly, each of you is a hero of today and of tomorrow. You save lives every day.

Marketing Questions You Should Ask Yourself

Are you ready to market your company's product or service? Here are a few marketing questions to ask yourself to help distinguish yourself from competitors:

1.   Have you considered whether or not your brand distinctly displays your message and values?

2.   Has your brand been portrayed accurately in all media that it has been advertised in?

3. Are you aware of your target audience and the best way to target it and direct its attention toward your product?

4. Are you accurately following trends in your brand, as well as consumers' reactions?

5. Is your understanding of the many factors that consumers take into account when buying your products recent and up-to-date?

6. Do you have at least one clear message that your product delivers to the media?

7. Have you intertwined social media into your marketing techniques?

8. When it comes to marketing channels, are you considering new options and better choices for both your brand and your consumers?

9. Have you considered creating a phone app in order to better communicate with your consumers and advertise your product?

10. Does your product shine in a large marketplace?

11. Have you delivered a creatively engaging message?

12. Do consumers remember your product?

13. Has your message been portrayed in a distinct and clear tone?

14. Is there a considerable upward trend in your product's sales? If not, what are you doing incorrectly?

15. Do you regularly offer your consumers chances to provide their personal input?

16. Does your product have something of value to offer consumers?

17. Do your various sales offers and deals accurately display your product?

18. Are all your sales ideas and data integrated into your brand's advertisement?

19. Have you considered new ideas regarding sales?

20. In what ways are you able to directly communicate with your audience?

21. Are your consumers able to connect to you and your brand?

22. Is your website optimized to suit search engines?

23. Do you update your website regularly?

24. Do your advertisements display valuable content that engages the audience?

25. Is your website simply designed for all users' navigation ease?

26. Are you recording responses and trends in regard to your product?

27. Do you have a business plan for your product?

28. Are you changing aspects of your product to attract specific groups of buyers?

29. Have you offered your audience ways to contact your management in order to deal with problems?

30. Do you have a clear plan on how to deal with warranties and customer service?

Chapter 6

The Learning Process

Understand that as you navigate your way as a Nurse Entrepreneur, there is a process and there are steps to go through to be successful. I am reminded of a Quote by Ziz Ziglar that says "There is no elevator to success, you have to take the stairs.

- Mission—how to discover your mission—so that you will know why you are in business and how you can make a difference.

- Mind-set—how to reframe your mind-set—so that you can learn how to show your authentic self.

- Market—how to identify your target market so that you can find those ideal clients eager to do business with you.

- Message—how to craft your marketing message so that you can have a clear and compelling answer to the question "What do you do?"

- Money—do you have enough money to fund the project?

- Model—how to decide on your business model—so that you can decide how to package and price your services to bring the best value for your clients and payment for your expertise.

- Mix—how to customize your market mix so you choose marketing strategies that work for your personality, strength, and business.

- Mastery—how to build your business mastery skills so that you can learn how to implement systems.

- making it work—how to use all seven steps of this business success strategy so that you can build a profitable long-term business.

Chapter 7

Leadership Tips and Summary

Every one of us was given a certain measure of a dream, and it is up to us to decide what to do and how we utilize it. You were called to this profession to be a nurse—that is, to care for, to treat, to nurture, and to educate. Whether you are happy with your current employment or not, you must evaluate your decision to become a nurse and question what values you sought during that process. After thirty years in this profession, I can attest to the many changes in the nursing field. What I want you to leave with is that regardless of the change that is occurring within the health-care field, you still have the power within you to affect others and change lives through your capacity as a nurse—even if that means reinventing your career. There is no cookie-cutter job requirement that defines what a true nurse is. Yes, we all have medical training and our respective degrees and certifications, but at the heart of it all, the ends of making a difference in people's lives are the same, even if the means through which we go about this goal are different. If you have considered using your talents and licensures in another capacity besides the traditional bedside nurse, the time to act is now! Legislations such as the Affordable Care Act have set the arena to bring forth a great change in the health-care system as we know it. Baby boomers are aging, and there will be calls to action within our field in many areas that were previously unforeseen. Whatever you decide, do not let fear of failure hinder your decision. You have the potential for greatness, and you can exercise your call to nursing in a plethora of ways.

If Entrepreneurship is your passion, now is the time to start. Follow your passion and your business and get ready to launch. For more information on starting your Nursing or your Health Care business, please contact the Author-

Eva M Francis RN, MSN, CCRN

www.EvaMFrancis.com

info@brillianthealthcaregroup.com

Yours in good health,

Eva M. Francis.

About the Author

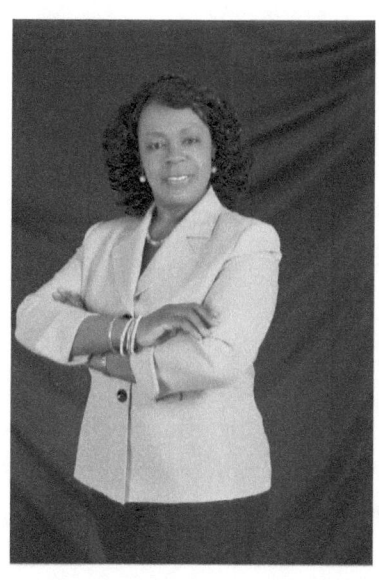

Eva Francis

South Florida-based Eva Francis is a registered nurse and an accomplished nursing and hospital administrator with more than two decades of experience in the healthcare industry. She received her bachelor's and master's degrees in nursing from Florida Atlantic University. Eva worked as a nurse executive, leading the company in executing business plans, facility and clinical program development, staff and leadership development, and healthcare training.

Her ultimate goal is to raise the bar in the field of nursing and health care, so as a health care consultant, inspirational speaker, leadership coach, and reinvention strategist, she conducts seminars, conferences, workshops, coaching and training on providing excellent service and leadership and business development. In addition, Eva partners with Florida Board of Nursing, American Heart Association, and healthcare organizations to transform the culture throughout the healthcare system.

Also, she is the author of Divine Health & Wellness Matter. She is the founder and owner of Brilliant Healthcare & Leadership Inc. that provides training and leadership and business development services to nurses, physicians, and other Healthcare providers. Her track record shows how she led organizations toward improved business processes, effective clinical operations, and quality patient care services, measures, and overall hospital operations.

Through her innovative techniques, Eva delivers, promotes and activates both energetic and engaged healthcare and business environments through her successful series of workshops. Also, she mentors nurse leaders, ensuring that the staff is provided with adequate training in executing processes and procedures set by management, along with meeting and exceeding industry standards.

Eva speaks to healthcare professionals and others on topics such as service excellence in healthcare, transforming culture to improve patient experience, helping leaders thrive in a challenging healthcare climate, emergency department excellence and taking your ER to the next level, and finding your passion through reinvention.

She was named Nurse of the Year and received the Humanitarian Award from the University Of Miami Hospital (formerly Cedars Medical Center). Eva strongly believes that "age does not define you. It's just a number, and one should not use their age to determine their success or their progress in life." She believes in working hard, embracing your dreams, consistently seeking to discover your purpose, and walking in it.

Having authored two e-books, she feels fulfilled knowing that she is touching lives and serving others in a bigger and brighter way through her gifts and talents. Eva said she was called to be more, have more, and give more.

Eva now helps healthcare professionals and leaders to elevate their personal and professional lives so that they can live a more fulfilling and successful life.

Index